IMPROVING LUNG HEALTH IN 30 DAYS

Pulmonary Rehabilitation Plan for COPD, Emphysema, Fibrosis, Bronchiectasis, and More

By Robert Redfern

Learn more about Pulmonary Rehabilitation, a plan
that will improve symptoms noticeably with
the potential for long-term relief.

ABOUT THE AUTHOR

Robert Redfern – Your Personal Health Coach
www.goodhealthhelpdesk.com

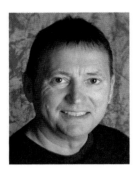

Robert Redfern was born in January 1946. He has helped thousands of people to date in more than 24 countries by providing online health guidance and resources in books, radio interviews, and TV interviews to share his nutritional discoveries. His new book series starts with the Healthier Heart e-book and is designed to bring all of his health knowledge into one user-friendly format that anyone can understand when pursuing health recovery.

Robert became interested in health when he and his wife Anne began to take charge of their lifestyle in the late 80s. Robert had not paid much attention to his health until 1986, despite Anne's loving influence. It wasn't until Robert's parents Alfred and Marjorie died prematurely in their 60s that he was forced to re-examine his lifestyle choices. Robert and Anne embraced a new health philosophy as they examined the health community, medical treatments, and common health issues.

After researching the root cause of disease, they discovered that diet and lifestyle choices were the two most pivotal factors that contribute to overall health and well-being. Robert and Anne decided to make major changes in their diet and lifestyle, while utilizing **HealthPoint™** acupressure. The changes that they saw were exceptional.

> In addition to improved health, Robert and Anne both look and feel like they have more vitality than they did decades before they started their new health plan. Currently, Robert, 68, and Anne continue to make healthy choices to live energetically and youthfully, based on a foundation of Natural Health.

Dedication:

For Marjorie Redfern, my mother, who died prematurely from Bronchiectasis and COPD. Her story has helped me to guide thousands of people in the rehabilitation of lung disease.

£4.99 / $6.99

ROBERT REDFERN – YOUR PERSONAL HEALTH COACH
Provides step-by-step guidance on:

IMPROVING LUNG DISEASE WITH SCIENTIFICALLY PROVEN PULMONARY REHABILITATION TO SUPPORT LUNG HEALTH

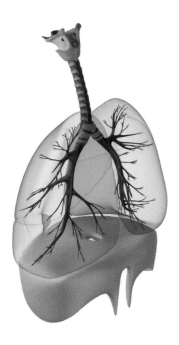

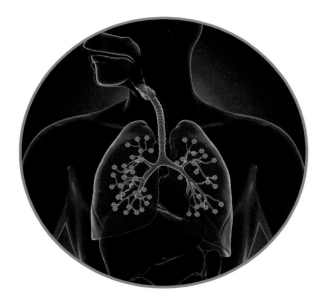
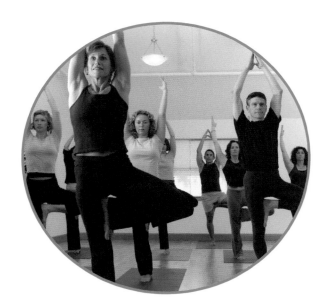

Publication printed in the United Kingdom.

Publisher's Note: This book is not intended to diagnose any disease or offer medical advice. The intention of the book is only to provide information for the reader so that they can make healthy lifestyle choices.

Warning: Some of the information in this book may contradict advice from your physician; nonetheless, content is based on the science of natural health.

CONTENTS

YOUR COMMITMENT PLAN FOR IMPROVED LUNG HEALTH

	ACTION	DATE
Commit	To a lifestyle of healthy choices	
Commit	To drinking more water: 8-10 glasses per day	
Commit	To spending more time in the sun: 20 minutes per day, except when contraindicated	
Read	Improving Lung Health in 30 Days	
Order	Supplements to support my healing action plan	
Plan	Create a menu plan through **ReallyHealthyFoods.com**	
Start	Breathing rehabilitation exercises	
Start	Lung rehabilitation exercises	
Start	Acupressure point massage	
Reread	Improving Lung Health in 30 Days	
Review	Supplements to support my healing action plan	
Review	Water intake commitment	
Review	Menu plan commitment	
Review	Breathing exercise commitment	
Review	Lung rehabilitation exercises	
Review	Sun exposure commitment, except when contraindicated	
Review	Acupressure massage commitment	
Recommit	To a lifestyle of healthy choices	
Recommit	To Improving Lung Health in 30 Days	
Recommit	To taking supplements to support my healing action plan	
Recommit	To drinking more water	
Recommit	To my menu plan	
Recommit	To breathing rehabilitation exercises	
Recommit	To lung rehabilitation exercises	
Recommit	To healthy sun exposure, except when contraindicated	
Recommit	To acupressure point massage	

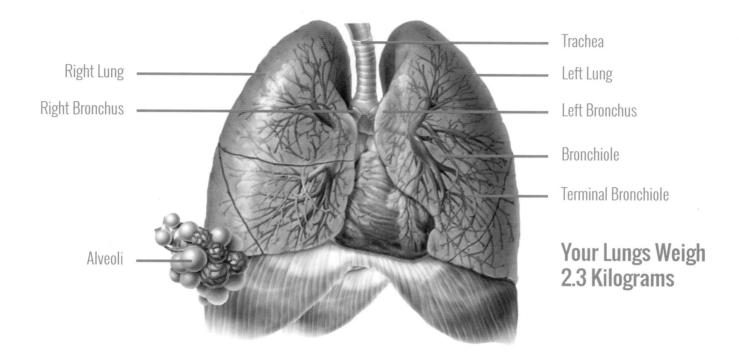

Right Lung

Right Bronchus

Alveoli

Trachea

Left Lung

Left Bronchus

Bronchiole

Terminal Bronchiole

**Your Lungs Weigh
2.3 Kilograms**

Understanding the Lungs

The lungs are respiratory organs that offer life and health in the form of oxygen. They also expel carbon dioxide as a waste byproduct. Portions of the lungs will warm air as it is inhaled and purify it of dust particles. In your body, there are two lungs:

1. **Left Lung:** Divided in two different lobes.
2. **Right Lung:** Divided in three different lobes.

▸ The lungs hold approximately 1500 miles (2400 km) of airways, containing 300-500 million alveoli (air sacs).

Alveoli in the lungs have a total surface area equal to half a tennis court. If you were to unwind all of the capillaries surrounding the alveoli, laying them end to end, they would measure at 620 miles long (992 km).

▸ The lungs as an organ weigh 5 pounds (2.3 kg), or 2.5 pounds each (1.1 kg each).

The lungs control respiration by exchanging air, allowing oxygen to be absorbed and waste gases to be pulled from the bloodstream. This process is called breathing. I recommend reading the breathing section on **page 33** to learn essential breathing exercises to support proper lung health.

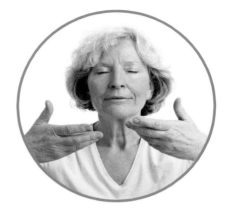

The nervous system is regulated by hormones to control breathing patterns by:

• **Increasing lung airflow**
• **Constricting lung airflow (mucus)**
• **Changing breathing patterns (related to stress or anxiety)**
• **Relaxing breathing patterns**

Lung capacity will depend on a number of factors, including:

• **Height**
• **Gender**
• **Altitude**
• **Smoking**

With age, the lungs shrink, often related to inflammation, poor nutrition, lack of use, and improper breathing patterns. Roughly 30% of all deaths are related to dysfunctional lungs, making it more important than ever to keep these organs in good health.

An average breath has a volume of 1 pint (500 mL). A typical respiratory rate for a resting adult is 10-20 breaths per minute with one third of each breath time used for inhalation.

Breathing patterns can be influenced by relaxation and anxiety. A person with lung disease may often breathe in an anxious pattern, further adding to their lung dysfunction.

Even a small amount of high-intensity exercise can noticeably improve lung capacity. The goal is to reduce breaths to roughly 6 breaths per minute in a relaxed state. The average person will breathe in 11,000 L of air, made up of 21% oxygen, each day.

▸ **If you are suffering with a lung condition, make it your goal to beat this average using the Pulmonary Rehabilitation Plan.**

Examples of lung function tests:

• Spirometry: Will measure the volume and flow of inhaled and exhaled air.
• Peak Flow Meter: Will measure maximum expiration speed.
• OxyMeter: Will measure blood oxygen content.

You can use these lung function tests to measure the success of your Rehabilitation Plan based on this book.

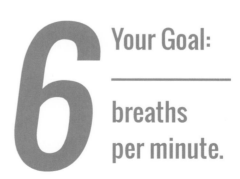

Your Goal:

6 breaths per minute.

Understanding Lung Diseases and Causes

Suffering from a lung or chest condition can be detrimental to the patient and their family. Many of these conditions are considered life-threatening and may require a lifetime of medications and doctors' visits without any improvement in health.

The Miracle Enzyme

Making lifestyle changes and taking an enzyme known as Serrapeptase (derived from the silkworm), along with other critical nutrients, can make a major difference in supporting lung rehabilitation. When the enzyme Serrapeptase is combined with other nutrients, it can help to clear scar tissue, mucus, and lung inflammation. The body can then begin to heal itself to repair damaged lung tissue and improve lung function.

When Serrapeptase is combined with other essential nutrients and healthy lifestyle choices, it can alleviate:

- Emphysema
- COPD
- Bronchitis
- Bronchiectasis
- Pulmonary Fibrosis
- Pneumoconiosis (Asbestosis and related dust diseases)
- Cystic Fibrosis
- Chronic Cough
- Bronchial Asthma
- Pulmonary Tuberculosis

▸ You can rely on this Miracle Enzyme to support lung health.
A healthy life is a happy life.

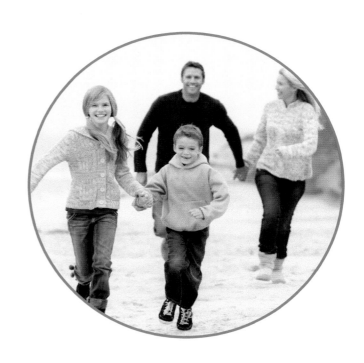

What Is COPD?

COPD (Chronic Obstructive Pulmonary Disease) affects millions of people in the Western world and is considered to be the fourth leading cause of death. COPD sufferers may have symptoms of emphysema and chronic bronchitis, as well as bronchial asthma. However, asthma is a condition that should be treated separately.

What causes it?

In many cases, COPD occurs secondary to chronic inflammation from high glycemic foods (high in sugar and starch), a nutritionally deficient diet, tobacco use, and pollution.

Though cystic fibrosis results from an alpha-1 antitrypsin deficiency, some rare types of bullous lung disease and bronchiectasis may also be contributing factors.

A. Normal lungs

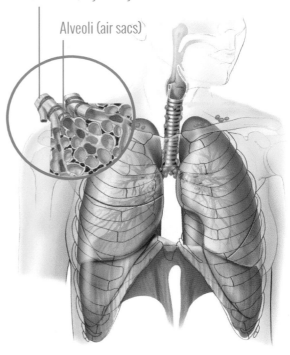

Bronchiole (tiny airways)

Alveoli (air sacs)

B. Lungs with COPD

Bronchioles lose their shape and become clogged with mucus.

Walls of alveoli are destroyed, forming fewer larger alveoli.

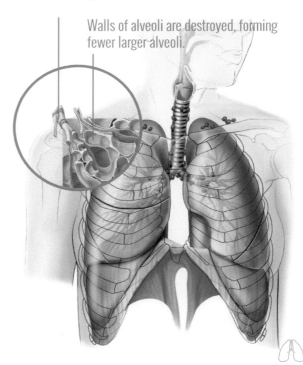

What Is Emphysema?

Emphysema occurs when the alveoli, or air sacs, in the lungs are destroyed; this is where oxygen in the air is replaced with carbon dioxide in the bloodstream. The walls of these air sacs are delicate and thin. When they are damaged, permanent holes are created in lower lung tissue. As air sacs are damaged, the lungs lose their ability to transfer as much oxygen to the blood, resulting in shortness of breath. The lungs will also have less elasticity. This may cause difficulty breathing, especially when exhaling, triggering even more breathing problems.

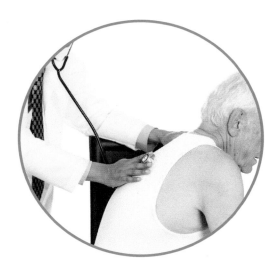

What causes it?

Emphysema isn't a condition that develops suddenly; it will occur gradually after long-term exposure to inflammation. The first indication comes with shortness of breath in physical activity. As the condition progresses, even a short walk can cause a bout of breathing issues. Chronic bronchitis may develop before emphysema occurs.

The main cause of emphysema is chronic inflammation related to:

- **Eating too many starchy foods**
- **Dairy foods**
- **Weak immune system**
- **Air pollution**
- **Smoking**

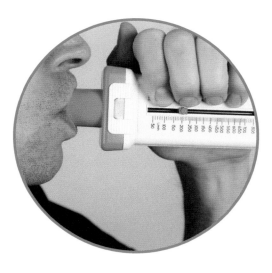

A diet that is deficient in vegetables and enzymes will also contribute to emphysema and increase the likelihood of infection.

▸ Remember, the first sign of emphysema is shortness of breath in physical activity.

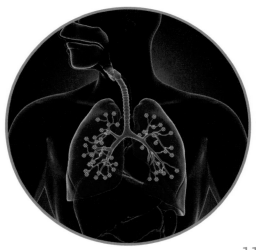

What Is Bronchitis?

Bronchitis occurs when the mucous membranes that transport air to the lungs become inflamed. Cases of bronchitis may be acute or chronic.

Acute bronchitis can start out as a cough and may be related to an acute, viral illness, like influenza or the common cold. Viruses are responsible for roughly 90% of acute bronchitis cases, compared to bacteria at less than 10%.

▸ **Chronic bronchitis is a type of COPD, characterized by a cough that lasts for three months or more a year for at least two years.**

Chronic bronchitis may be the result of recurrent airway injury related to inhaled irritants. For example, cigarette smoking is a common cause of chronic bronchitis, next to occupational exposure and air pollution.

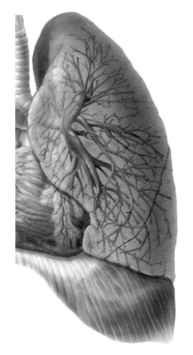

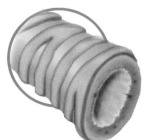

Normal bronchial tube

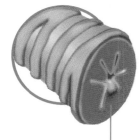

Inflamed lining of the bronchial tube

Thick mucus

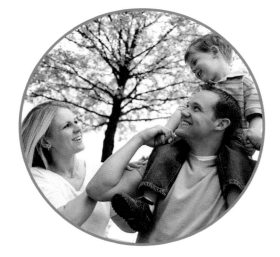

What Causes Bronchitis?

The main cause of bronchitis is chronic inflammation related to:

- **Eating too many starchy foods**
- **Dairy foods**
- **Weak immune system**
- **Air pollution**
- **Smoking**

A diet that is deficient in vegetables and enzymes will also contribute to bronchitis and increase the likelihood of infection.

What Is Pulmonary Fibrosis?

Fibrosis, including IPF, is the result of thickened or scarred lung tissue. Pulmonary fibrosis, Wegener's Granulomatosis, and Sarcoidosis all include fibrosis.

What Causes Pulmonary Fibrosis?

Pulmonary fibrosis may be the result of a number of factors, like:

- **Mineral deficiency, especially selenium and iodine**

- **Infections**

- **Chronic inflammation**

- **Environmental agents, like silica, asbestos, or certain gas exposure**

- **Ionizing radiation exposure, including radiation therapy to treat chest tumors**

- **Chronic health conditions, i.e. rheumatoid arthritis and lupus**

- **Some medications**

A condition called hypersensitivity pneumonitis causes lung fibrosis to develop after a heightened immune response when organic dust or occupational chemicals are inhaled. This condition most often occurs when contaminated dust containing fungi, bacteria, or animal products is inhaled.

Sometimes, fibrosis and chronic pulmonary inflammation can develop without any known cause. Many of these patients are diagnosed with idiopathic pulmonary fibrosis (IPF) that will not respond to medical treatment; other types of fibrosis, like non-specific interstitial pneumonitis (NSIP), may respond better to immunosuppressive therapy or immune balancing nutrients.

▸ **With either case, it's important to use the Pulmonary Rehabilitation Plan to clear up the condition completely or manage the health issue without the use of medication.**

A. Normal Lungs

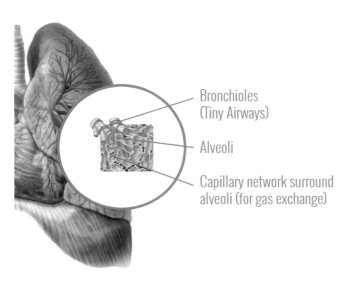

Bronchioles (Tiny Airways)

Alveoli

Capillary network surround alveoli (for gas exchange)

B. Lungs with Idiopathic Pulmonary Fibrosis (IPF)

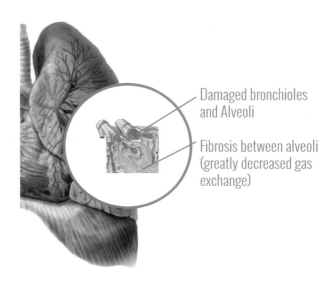

Damaged bronchioles and Alveoli

Fibrosis between alveoli (greatly decreased gas exchange)

What Is Bronchiectasis?

Bronchiectasis (brong-kee-ECK-tah-sis) is a rare lung condition that often occurs in infants and older children; adults can get bronchiectasis in some cases. Without any related complications, bronchiectasis isn't considered serious, but it can become a lifestyle issue when other health problems are present.

▸ **Bronchiectasis does not have a cure and can inhibit a normal lifestyle without the proper treatment.**

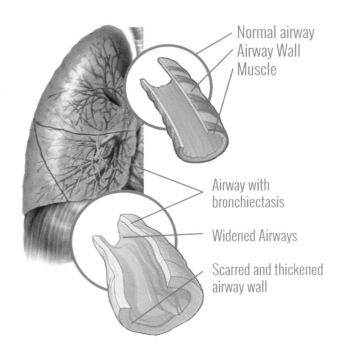

Normal airway
Airway Wall
Muscle

Airway with bronchiectasis

Widened Airways

Scarred and thickened airway wall

In bronchiectasis, bronchial tubes will become distended and enlarged to form pockets of infection. When the walls become damaged, it will impair the lungs' cleaning system. Tiny hairs (cilia) that line the bronchial tubes and filter germs, dust, and excess mucus are affected. When the cleaning system of the lungs is compromised, bacteria, mucus, and dust will build up. This breeds infection that is difficult to treat.

What Causes Bronchiectasis?

Bronchiectasis is the result of a number of infections that cause damage to the bronchial walls and cilia. Some people may be predisposed to the health condition due to a number of inherited or congenital deficiencies, including cystic fibrosis and immunological deficiency.

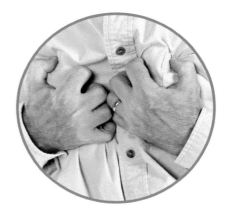

In rare cases, a genetic abnormality of the cilia may make a person more susceptible to bronchiectasis. Pneumonias caused by whooping cough and childhood measles may also trigger a predisposition to the condition by breaking down the walls of the bronchial tubes to allow pockets of infection to form.

If an obstruction presses on the inner bronchial tubes or blocks the outside of the bronchial tubes, it can also trigger bronchiectasis. In children, choking on a small object like a nut that gets lodged in the windpipe may block off an air tube. If this occurs, it will injure the wall of the tube and prevent air from passing. The bronchial tube below the obstruction will balloon out and collect infection and pus.

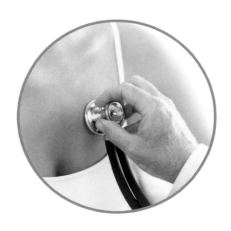

What Is Pneumoconiosis?
(Miner's Lung)

Pneumoconiosis includes asbestosis and other industrial/dust lung conditions, like Farmer's Lung, Berylliosis, Miner's Lung, Aritosis, Siderosis, and Stannosis.

What Causes Pneumoconiosis?

Pneumoconiosis occurs when the lungs are damaged from dust and other industrial materials. Fiber and asbestos dust can trigger asbestosis as the lungs scar to cause breathing issues and eventual heart failure due to lack of oxygen. Asbestosis is often associated with lung cancer, which may develop in an asbestos worker that also smokes cigarettes.

▸ **Risk increases 90 times in an asbestos worker that smokes compared to a non-smoker that works in an asbestos-free environment.**

Other dust diseases may include:

- **Berylliosis: After inhaling beryllium dust.**

- **Baritosis, Siderosis, and Stannosis: After inhaling barium sulphate, iron oxide (arc-welding fumes), and tin oxide respectively.**

- **Coal Worker's Pneumoconiosis: After inhaling coal dust.**

- **Farmer's Lung: After exposure to cereal, grain, or other industrial dust.**

Mesothelioma of the pleura is an asbestos related condition that is both serious and malignant, albeit rare. Compared to asbestosis, malignant pleural tumor mesothelioma may not be related to heavy asbestos fiber exposure.

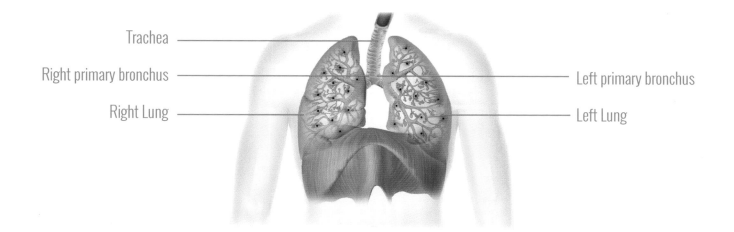

Trachea

Right primary bronchus

Right Lung

Left primary bronchus

Left Lung

What Is Cystic Fibrosis?

Cystic fibrosis (CF) is a genetic disorder that occurs in cells lining the pancreas, sweat glands, small intestine, and lungs. Mucus houses infection and leads to the destruction of lung tissue; it also interferes with gas exchange in the lungs. Mucus will prevent nutrient absorption in the small intestine by blocking pancreatic ducts that normally release digestive enzymes.

Cystic fibrosis is the most prevalent life-threatening genetic disease among Caucasians, though it can occur in all races and ethnicities. Cystic fibrosis will lead to malnutrition, weight loss, growth failure, and eventually, premature death.

With this condition, it's critical to improve nutrition and prevent chronic malnutrition symptoms like:

- **Being underweight**
- **Fat malabsorption**
- **Insufficient pancreatic function**
- **Abdominal pain**
- **Rectal prolapse**
- **Gut obstruction**
- **Heartburn**
- **Respiratory infection**
- **Pancreatitis**
- **Peptic ulcers**
- **Crohn's disease**
- **Liver disease**
- **Excessive mucus**

What Causes Cystic Fibrosis?

Cystic fibrosis is considered the most common hereditary genetic disease, possibly caused by a mineral deficiency. Cystic fibrosis worsens with a poor diet.

How Is Cystic Fibrosis Treated?

CF is a genetic disease that does not currently have a cure. This is why it's critical to follow a strict nutritional plan to improve health. The appropriate nutritional regimen for cystic fibrosis will depend on the progression of the disease; optimal nutrition is essential to support healthy growth and quality of life.

Health problems associated with cystic fibrosis may include:

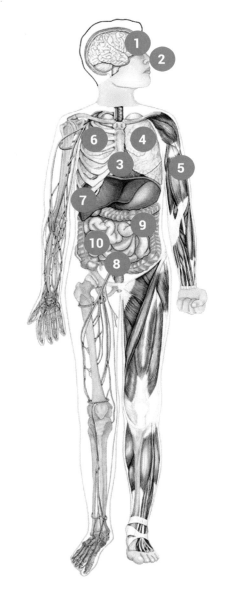

1. Sinus issues
2. Nose polyps
3. Enlarged heart
4. Recurring lung infections
5. Salty sweat
6. Difficulty breathing
7. Gallstones
8. Constipation
9. Abnormal pancreas function
10. Difficulty digesting food

What Is Chronic Cough?

If you have a cough that has lasted for over three weeks, it could be chronic. A health condition that is chronic means that it lasts for quite some time.

Ask yourself:

- Am I coughing up thick green or yellow phlegm?

- Am I wheezing or whistling when I breathe in?

▸ **Answering yes to either of those questions could mean that you need to see your doctor right away.**

What Causes Chronic Cough?

A virus is the main cause of chronic cough, in most cases. Smoking can also contribute to a cough that won't go away.

Chronic Cough and Allergies

Postnasal drip related to allergies can trigger a cough.

Postnasal drip means that mucus will run down the throat from the back of the nose. Postnasal drip related to allergies may be triggered by certain allergens that must be avoided, like:

- **Smoke**
- **Dust**
- **Mold**
- **Pollen**
- **Freshly cut grass**
- **Pets**
- **Some plants**
- **Room deodorizers**
- **Cleaning chemicals**
- **Chemical fumes**

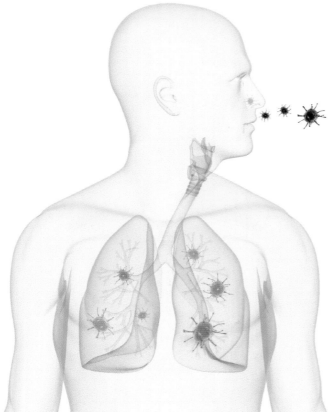
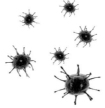

▸ **It's important to stop smoking as soon as possible.**

What Is Bronchial Asthma?

Asthma is a range of several related diseases with a number of causes. It is possible for asthma to be life threatening if it is only medicated, and the condition should be taken seriously.

If you have asthma, it's critical to:

1. **Take asthma seriously.**
2. **Start taking asthma medications.**
3. **Get help if asthma symptoms don't clear up.**
4. **Pay attention to asthma symptoms.**
5. **Come up with a plan to wean yourself off asthma medication and control the condition without the use of drugs; drugs have short and long-term side effects that can shorten your life.**

What Causes Bronchial Asthma?

The pharmaceutical industry would love for you to believe that asthma is triggered by dust mites, pollution, genetics, and more. This leaves you without any answers, forced to continue using asthma medication. The alternative viewpoint is that panic attacks and diet can trigger allergies; anxiety and the absence of friendly bacteria are contributing factors.

▸ Some people may be genetically predisposed to asthma, but this is not a life sentence. Proper rehabilitation can help to clear up asthma, even in these cases.

Common triggers of asthma include:

- **Allergies**
- **Infections**
- **Intense exercise**
- **Stress/anxiety/excitement**
- **Cold air**
- **Occupational dust/vapor**
- **Air pollution**
- **Cleaning products**
- **Drugs**

All of these asthma triggers cause inflammation. As a result, the asthma drug of choice is an anti-inflammatory steroid.

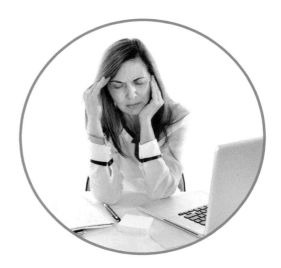

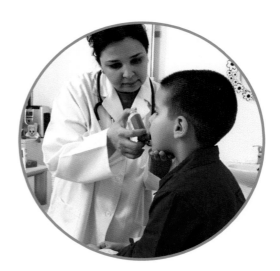

What Is Pulmonary Tuberculosis?

Pulmonary Tuberculosis is a contagious bacterial infection caused by TB, or Mycobacterium tuberculosis. Tuberculosis can easily spread from one person to another in the air. When a person has TB in their lungs or throat and laughs, coughs, sneezes, or talks, TB germs can spread into the air. If someone with a weak immune system inhales these germs, they could contract a tuberculosis infection.

What Causes Pulmonary Tuberculosis?

There is a difference between contracting a TB infection and having TB disease. A person with a healthy immune system that is infected with TB has TB bacteria living in their body. A healthy immune system will protect against these germs to prevent sickness.

If someone has TB disease and a weakened immune system, the disease can easily spread to other people. A person with tuberculosis needs to see a doctor as quickly as possible.

‣ Fortunately, it is fairly difficult to become infected with TB.

In most cases, you would have to spend a large amount of time with a person that has TB disease. TB may spread more easily between friends, family members, and coworkers. TB is spread in enclosed spaces over prolonged periods of time. In order for the disease to develop, tuberculosis bacteria must become pathogenic; a person under stress, eating a poor diet, or with a weakened immune system is more susceptible.

‣ Healthy people can become infected with TB, but they are less likely to get sick. It should be your number one goal to get and stay healthy.

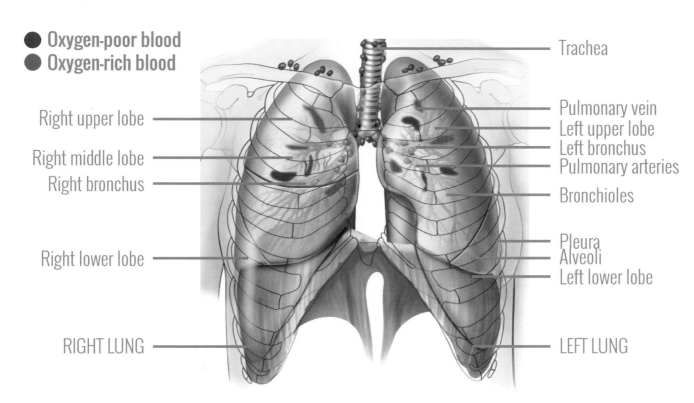

● Oxygen-poor blood
● Oxygen-rich blood

Right upper lobe
Right middle lobe
Right bronchus

Right lower lobe

RIGHT LUNG

Trachea

Pulmonary vein
Left upper lobe
Left bronchus
Pulmonary arteries

Bronchioles

Pleura
Alveoli
Left lower lobe

LEFT LUNG

Is It Possible to Reverse Lung Disease?

I prefer not to use the word "cure" when talking about lung disease since many are related to lifestyle problems, unless they are the result of a gene dysfunction. Cure is a popular medical buzzword, although the medical field cannot provide cures. (Many people argue that this is on purpose since it would put Big Pharma out of business.)

Every health condition has a cause. When you take away the underlying cause and follow the Pulmonary Rehabilitation Plan, your body will have the support it needs to repair itself, in many cases.

When you remove the cause and support your body with healthy lifestyle choices and nutrients, your lungs will often grow healthy again. You may call this a cure, but I believe it to be making healthy lifestyle choices.

Bronchitis, Bronchiectasis, Chronic Cough, Fibrosis, Emphysema, and Bronchial Asthma Causes

These conditions are caused by chronic inflammation related to factors like:

• Eating too many starchy foods
• Dairy foods
• Infection
• Lacking certain nutrients
• Smoking
• Improper breathing
• Pollution

In most cases, when you eliminate the cause, symptoms will clear up right away.

Pneumoconiosis, Asbestosis, and Related Dust Conditions Causes

These conditions are caused by chronic inflammation related to factors like:

• **Industrial contaminants**
• **Eating too many starchy foods**
• **Dairy foods**
• **Infection**
• **Lacking certain nutrients**
• **Smoking**
• **Improper breathing**
• **Pollution**

In most cases, when you eliminate the cause, symptoms will clear up right away. At the very least, they will be managed so that they are no longer a problem.

Cystic Fibrosis Causes

This condition is caused by chronic inflammation related to factors like:

• **Genetic dysfunction**
• **Eating too many starchy foods**
• **Dairy foods**
• **Infection**
• **Lacking certain nutrients**
• **Smoking**
• **Improper breathing**
• **Pollution**

In most cases, when you eliminate the cause, symptoms will clear up right away. At the very least, they will be managed so that they are no longer a problem.

▸ … transform your health with a balanced lifestyle and essential nutrients …

Essential Nutrients

According to research, these nutrients can manage or improve lung conditions in most cases:

Serrapeptase - Used to clear inflammation and scarring.

Curcumin - Used to clear inflammation and support tissue healing.

Ecklonia Cava - Seaweed extract supports lung healing.

Vitamin D3 - Supported by numerous studies to enhance lung and immune health and aid in recovery.

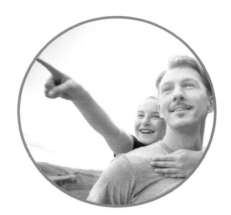

Oxygen Promoting Enzymes - Used to enhance the lungs' ability to clear CO2 and intake more oxygen.

Sodium Thiocyanate/Sodium Hypothiocyanite - Essential to support the body's defense against infection.

Food State Iodine Drops - Critical mineral to support all lung health issues, especially fibrosis.

EpiCor - Yeast extract used to balance the body's immune response.

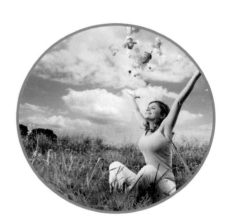

Selenium - Critical co-factor of iodine to support cellular regeneration and protection.

Essential Fatty Acids - Krill, Fish, or Hemp Oil, essential for all people.

Multi Vitamin and Mineral Complex - To supplement any missing nutrients.

Digestive Enzymes - Essential pancreatic support, especially after eating cooked foods.

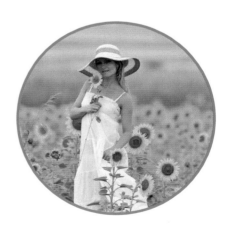

Probiotics - Friendly bacteria will support beneficial gut flora, especially after taking antibiotics.

Vitamin E (Mixed Tocotrienols) - Essential for all lung health conditions, especially Cystic Fibrosis.

What If the Medical Industry Doesn't Support My Recovery?

The drug model in the medical industry supports the monopoly of the pharmaceutical industry: the GMC in the UK and the AMA in the USA, which affect the health of all people. These organizations turn a profit in treating sickness, although they don't support long-term health and recovery.

Instead, they work with a patented drug model that allows them to charge unreasonable prices for a lifetime of medications that may provide some relief but often speed up death. These drugs aren't designed to improve health. In the US, the monopoly is protected by the FDA and in the UK, by the MHRA. Powerful politicians are paid by these organizations to create laws that continue the vicious cycle of disease management monopoly.

▸ **Yet when you follow the Pulmonary Rehabilitation Program to the letter, you can see results within weeks.**

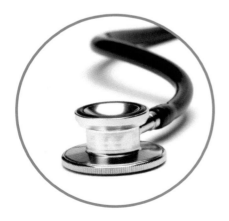

What Is Pulmonary Rehabilitation?

Pulmonary Rehabilitation has more than 30 years of research behind it and is defined as:

- Pulmonary Rehabilitation (or pulmonary rehab) is a type of rehabilitation treatment geared toward sick patients with chronic respiratory issues and decreased pulmonary function, despite medical treatment.

- This program will teach you how to breathe easier to improve quality of life through treatment, physical activity, information, and coaching.

- This is a personalized program that integrates education, support, and therapy to help you reach the maximum function permitted by your condition.

Pulmonary Rehabilitation was first documented by Charles Denison in 1895. Since that time, hundreds of supporting studies have been published. Granted, the pharmaceutical industry chooses to overlook these studies and prefers that patients stay stuck in their rut, dependent on medication.

▸ **Now you have learned there is a better way.**

In the following pages, we will detail the Pulmonary Rehabilitation Program that can provide results in weeks, when it is followed carefully.

"It will be a good day when the information doctors need to prescribe is made available from an independent body that has a legal responsibility to ensure the efficacy and safety of drugs."

Your Pulmonary Rehabilitation Plan for Lung Health

10 Steps for Long-Term Health Recovery

This self-recovery protocol can be used for any lung health issue, in most cases.

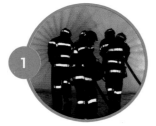

1 Clear inflammation and facilitate healing.

Eat really healthy foods. **6**

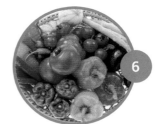

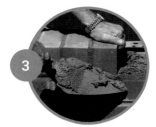

2 Supplement missing nutrients.

Stay active daily. **7**

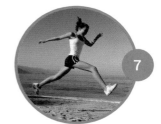

3 Boost the immune system.

Learn proper breathing. **8**

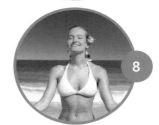

4 Drink more water.

Stimulate acupressure points. **9**

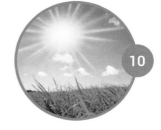

5 Cut out unnatural foods.

Get more sun exposure. **10**

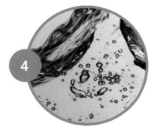

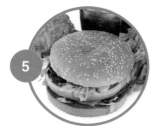

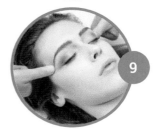

It's almost impossible not to see significant lung health changes after applying many of the points in this 10 Step Plan. You can clear up numerous symptoms and may see a full recovery, in many cases.

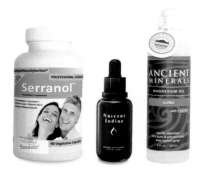

To find out more about the suggested formulas, please see **page 35.**

1. Clear Inflammation and Facilitate Healing.

#1 Lung Health - <u>Basic Plan</u>

Serranol™ - **Provides 80,000 IU of SerraEnzyme Serrapeptase, 250mg of CurcuminX4000, 50mg of Ecklonia Cava, and 1000 IU of Vitamin D3.**

Nascent Iodine Drops - **Offers an atomic form of consumable iodine as a supplement, just as natural as iodine used in the body.**

Magnesium OIL Spray ULTRA - **Magnesium Oil now formulated with OptiMSM® to enhance absorption.**

2. Supplement Missing Nutrients.

#2 Lung Health - <u>Advanced Plan</u>

Serranol™ - **Provides 80,000 IU of SerraEnzyme Serrapeptase, 250mg of CurcuminX4000, 50mg of Ecklonia Cava, and 1000 IU of Vitamin D3.**

Nascent Iodine Drops - **Offers an atomic form of consumable iodine as a supplement, just as natural as iodine used in the body.**

Magnesium OIL Spray ULTRA - **Magnesium Oil now formulated with OptiMSM® to enhance absorption.**

DIP Daily Immune System - **Formulated with proven ingredients to fight infection, protect against immune responses to allergens, and support immune health.**

OxySorb - **Liquid enzyme aids in oxygen absorption and clears CO2 in the body.**

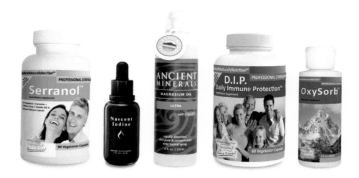

3. Boost the Immune System.

#3 Lung Health - Ultimate Plan

Serranol™ - Provides 80,000 IU of SerraEnzyme Serrapeptase, 250mg of CurcuminX4000, 50mg of Ecklonia Cava, and 1000 IU of Vitamin D3.

Nascent Iodine Drops - Offers an atomic form of consumable iodine as a supplement, just as natural as iodine used in the body.

Magnesium OIL Spray ULTRA - Magnesium Oil now formulated with OptiMSM® to enhance absorption.

DIP Daily Immune System - Formulated with proven ingredients to fight infection, protect against immune responses to allergens, and support immune health.

OxySorb - Liquid enzyme aids in oxygen absorption and clears CO2 in the body.

Prescript Assist - World Leading Soil Based Probiotic, the only formula available with scientifically proven studies.

ActiveLife 90 - Potent liquid vitamins and minerals formula; 300% more absorbent compared to tablets.

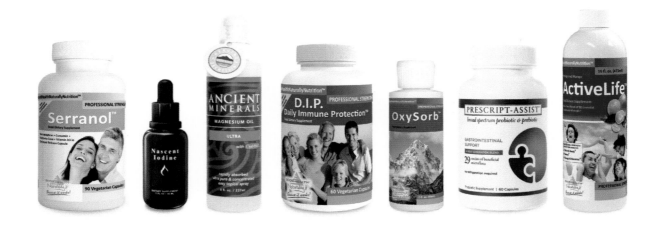

Optional - But Highly Recommended for At Least 1 to 2 Months

A. Ultimate Immune Support Kit

1st Line (Thiocyanate) Immune System Support Kit

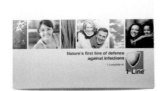

B. Digestive Enzymes

Essential Digestive Plus™

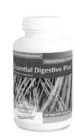

C. Vitamin E Mixed Tocotrienols (especially for Cystic Fibrosis)

Naturally Better Vitamin E

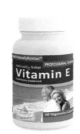

D. Krill Oil

The Krill Miracle

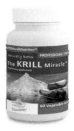

4. Drink More Water.

Drink at least 6-8 glasses of RO filtered or distilled water each day; add a generous pinch of baking soda to each glass.

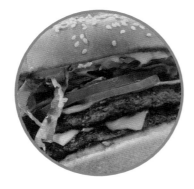

5. Cut Out Unnatural Foods.

Cut out starchy carbohydrates altogether, i.e. pastries, cookies, breads, breakfast cereals, pasta, and potatoes, as well as processed foods and milk products.

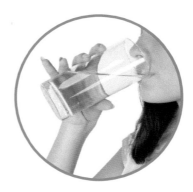

Note: Don't eat turnips, parsnips, and rice, except for small portions of wild rice, brown rice, and sweet potatoes/yams.

6. Eat Really Healthy Foods.

Make sure to eat some of these foods every two hours for the first few months of recovery:

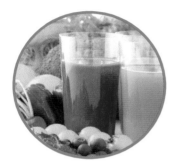

Eat 9-14 servings of fresh or frozen vegetables each day: try them in soups, steamed, stir-fried, juiced, etc. Eat 50% raw, juiced vegetables (preferably organic) and use the pulp to make soup. Blended veggies promote easier digestion.

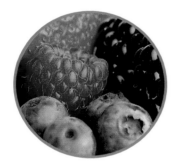

Eat 5 servings of dark-skinned fruits (like cherries, red grapes, blueberries, etc.) that are rich in antioxidants each day.

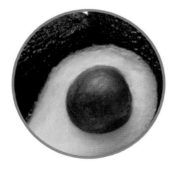

Remember that avocados are a number one superfood with almost a complete spectrum of nutrients. If they are readily available in your area, try to eat at least two a day to promote health recovery. Avocados support all lung health issues, heart disease, and even cancer recovery.

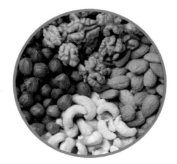

Eat 5 servings of nuts, beans, and seeds (soaked, mashed nuts and seeds).

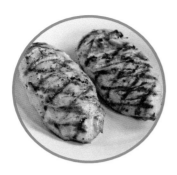

Eat pasture-fed chicken and other meats, only a few servings per week. Grass-fed meat is recommended above corn or grain-fed meat sources.

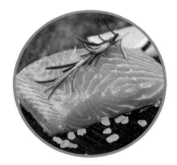

Eat a minimum of 3-4 servings of oily fish each week, if you eat fish. Choose a variety of healthy fish like mackerel, sardines, salmon, etc. Canned fish is a nutritious option, although wild caught fish is recommended.

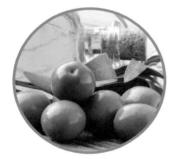

Add healthy oils to your favorite foods, like krill, omega 3, hemp, coconut, and olive oils.

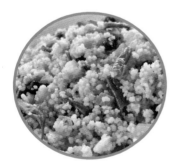

Pair with healthy carbohydrate alternatives, like amaranth, quinoa, buckwheat, and chai and millet seeds. You can also try couscous, if you aren't allergic to gluten protein (celiac disease).

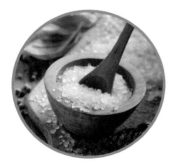

Add 3-5 teaspoons of sea or rock salt, depending on the heat and your body mass, to water or food each day. Remember that sea or rock salt does not contain the important mineral iodine, which is why it is recommended to use Nascent Iodine in your Rehabilitation Plan.

Which vegetables to eat

Note: Not all vegetables listed are available in every country.

- Artichoke
- Asian Vegetables Sprouts (Wheat, Barley, Alfalfa, etc)
- Asparagus
- Avocado
- Broad Beans
- Cabbage (various types)
- Dandelion Leaves
- Dried Peas
- Fennel
- Garden Peas
- Garlic
- Kale
- Lettuce (Kos and various types)
- Mangetout Peas
- Mushrooms
- Petit Pois Peas
- Runner Beans
- Seaweed all types (Kelp, Wakame, Noni, etc)
- Sugar Snap Peas
- Beetroot
- Broccoli
- Brussel Sprouts
- Capsicum
- Carrots
- Cauliflower
- Celeriac
- Choko
- Cucumber
- Eggplant (Aubergine) Kale
- Kohlrabi
- Kumara
- Okra
- Onions (Red and White)
- Radishes
- Silver Beet
- Spinach
- Squash
- Zucchini (Courgettes)

Which fruits to eat

Note: Not all fruits listed are available in every country.

- Apple
- Apricot
- Avocado
- Blackberries
- Blackcurrants
- Bilberries
- Blueberries
- Cherries
- Cherimoya
- Dates
- Damsons
- Durian
- Figs
- Gooseberries
- Grapes
- Grapefruit
- Kiwi fruit
- Limes
- Lychees
- Mango
- Nectarine
- Orange
- Pear
- Plum/Prune (dried Plum)
- Pineapple
- Pomegranate
- Raspberries
- Western raspberry (blackcap)
- Rambutan
- Salal berry
- Satsuma
- Strawberries
- Tangerine

Really Healthy Food Pyramid: *Garden of Eden*

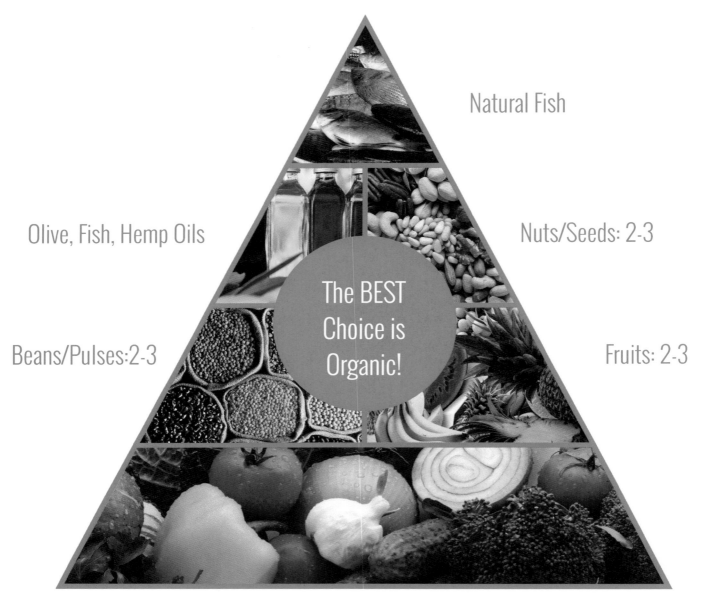

Natural Fish

Olive, Fish, Hemp Oils

Nuts/Seeds: 2-3

The BEST Choice is Organic!

Beans/Pulses:2-3

Fruits: 2-3

Vegetables (excluding root): 8-12 servings a day
1/2 raw veggies: salads, etc.

7. Stay Active Daily.

There are two recommended ways to get your body back into shape, beyond rigorous activities like swimming and cycling recommended by exercise enthusiasts. You are welcome to include these activities later on in your Rehabilitation Plan, if desired.

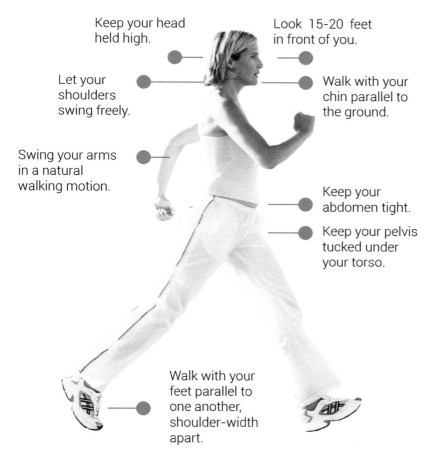

Keep your head held high.

Look 15-20 feet in front of you.

Let your shoulders swing freely.

Walk with your chin parallel to the ground.

Swing your arms in a natural walking motion.

Keep your abdomen tight.

Keep your pelvis tucked under your torso.

Walk with your feet parallel to one another, shoulder-width apart.

Walking is one simple way to build up your activity level at 3-5 miles per day. Walk with a brisk, purposeful gait in a long stride that is comfortable for you. Pump your hands from chest to waist level with each stride you take.

As your fitness level improves, feel free to incorporate weights, like wrist weights. It may be difficult for you to use weights as you begin if your lungs are weak; if exercise proves difficult, you can lie down to make exercise easier.

Start by lying down in a comfortable place, like a firm bed after waking up in the morning. Bring your knee to chest level and alternate with the other knee. Continue this motion as many times as possible as you keep count. Perform this exercise every day and set goals to increase the number of repetitions and the speed each week. This exercise should be performed with enough intensity to increase your heart rate and work your lungs. As you improve your count and speed, you can begin walking and building fitness from there.

The second recommended way to strengthen your lungs is to build up exercise to a maximum of two minutes, six times a day. You can choose any cardiovascular exercise you prefer, like running in place, jumping jacks, or skipping, as long as it works your lungs and heart at maximum capacity. When you exercise at maximum exertion, your heart, lungs, and connected muscles will naturally grow stronger to improve lung health.

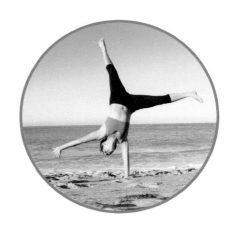

Physical activity is essential to your Pulmonary Rehabilitation Plan.

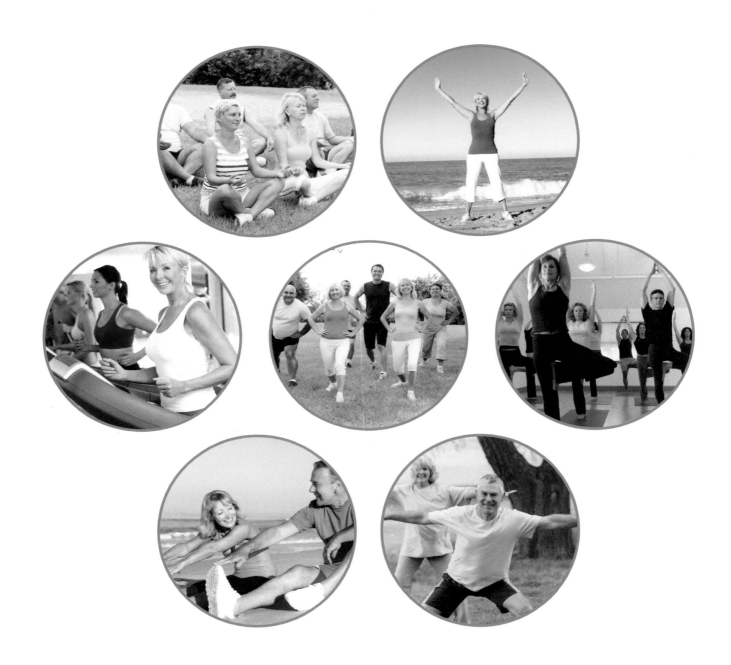

8. Learn Proper Breathing.

Breathing properly is critical since oxygen is the foundation of overall health. There are two types of breathing:

1. **Anxious Breathing: In the chest.**
2. **Relaxed Breathing: In the diaphragm or stomach area**.

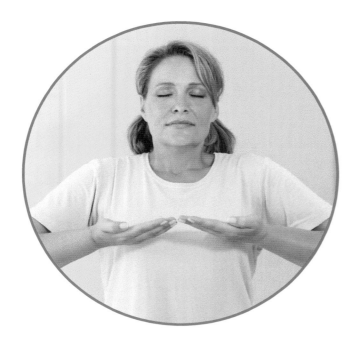

How to Breathe Correctly

The easiest way to relearn correct breathing is to lie flat on your back on the floor on a mat or blanket or on a firm bed. Place a small weighted object on your belly button, like a heavy book. Take a deep breath in through your nose so that the book rises as your stomach, or diaphragm, fills with air. Hold this deep breath for a count of 4 and then release through your nose so that your stomach deflates. Use this process to release any tension as you exhale and repeat. In the exercise, your chest should not move to indicate relaxed, stress-free breathing.

Practice this low-stress breathing exercise again and again as you lie down. Once you have mastered the rhythm of the calming breath, you can start to try the exercise while standing. Initially, you may feel dizzy as you intake more and more fresh oxygen, but it's still important to practice the exercise whenever you can.

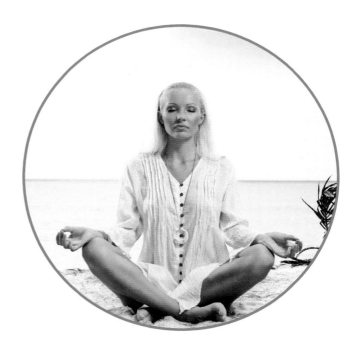

The first type of breathing in the chest is related to a stress response and includes hormones like cortisol. This stressful breathing should only be temporary since it is related to a fight-or-flight response that causes hormones to release to relax breathing. If stressful breathing grows chronic, the body will retain carbon dioxide and cortisol to affect healthy functioning systems. Stress breathing will also cause the immune system to weaken, leaving it susceptible to infection.

Make it your number one goal to retrain your body to breathe in a relaxed, healthy manner. This will clear out carbon dioxide and cortisol. When carbon dioxide builds up in your bloodstream, it will destroy a substance called hemoglobin that the blood uses to transport oxygen throughout the body. This is why it's especially important to focus on relaxed breathing that comes from the diaphragm.

9. Stimulate Acupressure Points.

Another critical component in your Pulmonary Rehabilitation Plan is to relax breathing by stimulating the main acupressure point, known as **Cv17** in Chinese acupuncture. It is located in a hollow in the sternum in the center of the chest; it falls in the center of the line traced from nipple to nipple across the chest. Massage this hollow with your finger gently or stimulate it with an electronic stimulator that will simulate actual acupuncture. I recommend the **HealthPoint™** device for this purpose. You can find more information on **page 40.**

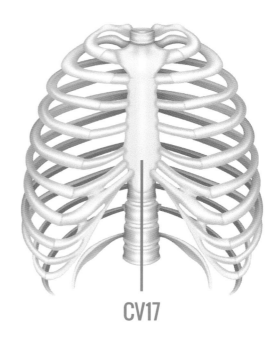

CV17

10. Get More Sun Exposure

An essential vitamin to support your overall health is vitamin D3. You can find a large dose of vitamin D3 in the recommended supplement on **page 35**, but it's still critical to get some natural vitamin D from sun exposure

The sun is the source of life. Unfortunately, myths have been circulated in the health community that the sun is an enemy that we must stay away from at all costs. Even worse, many health professionals recommend slathering your body in toxic chemicals every time you go out in the sun.

Of course, I'm not recommending lying in the sun for 6 hours at once on the first hot day of the year. It's essential to build up the skin's tolerance to sun exposure over several weeks for natural protection. By the time that hot summer days come around, you will be able to tolerate a greater amount of natural sun exposure.

Recommendations for sun exposure:

A: *Expose as much skin as you can to the sun each day, such as on your morning walk.*

-

B: *Build up your sun exposure gradually from spring to summer seasons.*

-

C: *Try to stay out of the sun in midday without a cover-up; a cover-up is preferred to sunscreen.*

-

D: *If you do use sunscreen or sun cream, purchase organic products instead of chemical-based, name-brand creams.*

-

E: *It's important to remember that the sun is your friend and sunshine can be enjoyed in moderation!*

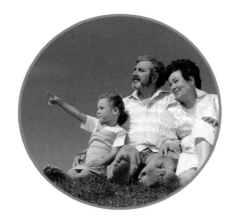

How to Clear Inflammation and Facilitate Healing

A Formula to Clear Inflammation, Mucus, and Scarring

Super Nutrient Serranol™

- **Serrapeptidase** (technically Serriatia Peptidase) is a diverse proteolytic enzyme that will dissolve non-living tissue, including blood clots, cysts, scarring, plaque, fibrin, and all types of inflammation, without causing harm to living tissue in the body. Serrapeptidase can be used to enhance your overall well-being, ease inflammation, and support health to benefit the lungs, joints, digestive tract, colon, arteries, and any other areas of blockage/inflammation.

- **Curcumin** is praised as one of the best natural, anti-inflammatory herbs. It can stimulate glutathione in the body to guard healthy cells and tissues against inflammation, while moderating the immune system. Curcumin is also known for its antiviral, antifungal, and antibacterial properties.

- **Ecklonia** has been used by the Asian population for centuries as a type of edible brown algae called Ecklonia Cava Extract. It is harvested off the coast of China, Korea, and Japan; studies support that ECE offers a wide range of health benefits.

- **Vitamin D3** is an essential vitamin to support immune health. Cells in the immune system are made up of vitamin D3 receptors. If there is a deficiency in vitamin D3, it will weaken the immune system and leave the body susceptible to infection. Unfortunately, vitamin D3 deficiency is becoming far too common amongst all age groups since our culture spends far less time in the sun. This valuable vitamin cannot be stored by the body, so daily supplementation is necessary for immune health.

Ingredients:

- SerraEnzyme Serrapeptase® 80,000iu
- Curcumin X4000 250mg
- Ecklonia Cava Extract (Seanol®) 50mg
- Vitamin D3 1000iu

Dosage:

Take 2 capsules, 3 times per day, 30 minutes before eating a meal with water, and reduce to 1 x 3 after a good relief.

Nascent Iodine

Nascent Iodine is entirely different from typical iodine found in a denser state, often sold over-the-counter as an antiseptic, labeled as atomized iodine tri-chloride, or added to potassium iodide so that it is liquid-soluble. Nascent Iodine is easily consumable iodine found in the atomic rather than the molecular form. It offers noticeable benefits in immune and thyroid support, as well as improved metabolism, detoxification, energy, and more.

Ingredients:

- Iodine (in its atomic form) 400 mcg

Dosage:

Take 4 x 4 drops per day in 25ml of water, swish around the mouth for 30 seconds then swallow. Build over 2 weeks up to 10 x 4 until well and then slowly reduce back to 4 x 4. Note that Iodine needs a supplement containing selenium to activate it such as ActiveLife 90 or Daily Immune Protection.

Ancient Minerals Magnesium Oil Ultra

Ancient Minerals Magnesium Oil Ultra is a cutting-edge formulation that maximizes the one-of-a-kind benefits of magnesium and MSM working in synergy together. Ancient Minerals Magnesium Oil Ultra will provide enhanced magnesium ion uptake and improve cell membrane permeability. It offers benefits to calm inflammation, improve joint mobility, and ease pain.

Ingredients:

- 1.6g elemental magnesium per fl oz.
- 3.6g of MSM (OptiMSM®) per fl oz.

Dosage:

Spray liberally onto the chest, back, and arm muscles to cover a wide area for absorption. Take regularly during the first 3-4 months of use to fully restore cellular magnesium levels.

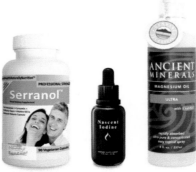

How to Supplement Missing Nutrients

Enzyme Formula to Promote Oxygen Absorption, Best for Breathing Difficulties

OxySorb

Lung health issues often cause the side effect of poor breathing, which can create even more problems by compromising oxygen/carbon dioxide exchange. This will worsen as the hemoglobin used in the body to transport essential oxygen is destroyed when carbon dioxide levels rise in the bloodstream. OxySorb offers a formulation made from seaweed extract to support the body's ability to clear carbon dioxide and transport oxygen more efficiently for overall health and recovery.

Ingredients:

- Tris Amino
- Norwegian Seaweed Extract
- Citric Acid
- Natural Kiwi Flavour

Dosage:

Take about 20 drops in the mouth, swish around for at least 30 seconds and then swallow. Repeat this process a minimum of twice a day and any time you need respiratory support.

Daily Immune Protection (D.I.P.)

One way to fight infection is by taking a formula created to balance immune health. D.I.P. will not kill existing infection, but it can help to prevent new infection from developing and reduce allergic reactions.

- **EpiCor®** - Potent antioxidant with an ORAC (Oxygen Radical Absorption Capacity) value at 52,500/100g, making it a highly beneficial free radical scavenger. EpiCor® has years of research and development to back it; it is considered an essential supplement to boost immune health.

- **ExSelen®** - The body depends on the essential trace mineral selenium, although it can't produce it on its own. Selenium must be ingested in the diet or through a supplement. ExSelen® offers powerful, bio-available organic selenium with consistently high levels of selenomethionine guaranteed (the ideal form to provide the best absorption in the body). ExSelen® is a superior raw material with 15 years of research and 60 years of proprietary fermentation technology behind it. It works as a natural antioxidant to guard healthy cells from free radical damage and support balanced immune health. Selenium enhances the normal inflammatory response in the lungs and may offer benefits in thyroid, prostate, and breast health.

- **Vitamin D3** is indispensable to a healthy immune system. Cells within the immune system contain vitamin D3 receptors; if there is not enough vitamin D3 to bind to the receptors, the body's immune defense against infection will weaken. Vitamin D3 deficiency is unfortunately common as the body does not store it. Vitamin D3 must be replenished by taking a daily supplement, critical for robust immune health.

Ingredients:

- EpiCor® 500mg
- ExSelen® selenomethionine 100mcg
- Vitamin D3 1000iu

Formulated with other powerful ingredients like:

- Vitamin C (from Ascorbic Acid) 120 mg
- Zinc Glycinate Chelate 20% 5 mg
- Dimethylglycine HCL 250 mg
- Elderberry Fruit Extract 4:1 200 mg
- Larch Arabinogalactan Powder 200 mg
- Immune Assist - Micron Powder 80 mg
- Beta Glucan 1,3 (Glucan 85%) 60 mg

Dosage:

Take 1 capsule, twice per day with meals.

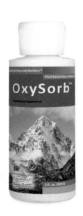
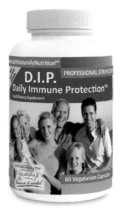

How to Boost Your Immune System

Active Life 90 Powerful Liquid Vitamins & Minerals

Active Life 90 Powerful Liquid Vitamins & Minerals comes in a convenient liquid formula to provide the essential vitamins and minerals that your body needs to thrive. This liquid supplement offers the best absorption and utilization within your body. It's 300% more absorbent than tablets!

Ingredients: Amount per Serving

Ingredient	Amount per Serving
Calories	39
Calcium (Tricalcium Phosphate, Citrate)	600mg
Choline Bitartrate	25mg
Chromium (Chromium Polynicotinate)	200mcg
Copper (Copper Gluconate)	2mg
Folic Acid (Vitamin B Conjugate)	500mcg
Inositol	50mg
Magnesium (Citrate Gluconate Concentrate)	300mg
Manganese (Manganese Gluconate)	10mg
Organic Seleniumethionine	200mcg
Potassium (Potassium Gluconate)	250mg
Vitamin A (Palmitate)	5000IU
Vitamin A (Beta Carotene)	5000IU
Vitamin B1 (Thiamine Mononitrate)	3mg
Vitamin B12 (Methylcobalamin)	6mcg
Vitamin B2 (Riboflavin)	3.4mg
Vitamin B3 (Niacinamide)	40mg
Vitamin B5 (Calcium Pantothenate)	20mg
Vitamin B6 (Pyridoxine Hydrochloride)	4mg
Vitamin C (Ascorbic Acid)	300mg
Vitamin D (Cholecalciferol)	400IU
Vitamin E (Alpha Tocopheryl Acetate)	60IU
Vitamin K (Phytonadione)	80mcg
Zinc (Oxide)	15mg
Ionic Trace Minerals	600mg
Phosphorus (Amino Acid Chelate)	190mg
Biotin	300mcg
Iodine (Potassium Iodine)	150mcg
Boron (Sodium Borate)	2mg
Molybdenum	75mcg
Chloride Concentrate	102mg
Amino Acid Complex	10mg
Aloe Vera Extract (200:1)	2mg

Dosage:

Take 15ml (1/2 fl. ounce) x 2 times per day with a little juice or water, with your breakfast and evening meals.

Prescript-Assist® (P-A)

Prescript-Assist® (P-A) provides a 3rd-generation formulation made up of 29 probiotic microflora "Soil-Based- Organisms (SBOs)" paired with a humic/fulvic acid prebiotic to improve SBO proliferation. Prescript-Assist's® microflora are categorized as Class-1 micro ecological units, the same that can naturally be found in a healthy gastrointestinal tract.

Ingredients

- *Proprietary blend of Leonardite*
- *Class I (beneficial microorganisms) : Anthrobacter agilis, Anthrobacter citreus, Anthrobacter globiformis, Anthrobacter luteus, Anthrobacter simplex, Acinetobacter calcoaceticus, Azotobacter chroococcum, Azotobacter paspali, Azospirillum brasiliense, Azospirillum lipoferum, Bacillus brevis, Bacillus marcerans, Bacillus pumilis, Bacillus polymyxa, Bacillus subtilis, Bacteroides lipolyticum, Bacteriodes succinogenes, Brevibacterium lipolyticum, Brevibacterium stationis, Kurtha zopfil, Myrothecium verrucaria, Pseudomonas calcis, Pseudomonas dentrificans, Pseudomonas flourescens, Pseudomonas glathei, Phanerochaete chrysosporium, Streptomyces fradiae, Streptomyces celluslosae, Streptomyces griseoflavus*

Dosage:

Take 1 capsule x 2 times a day (can be opened and mixed with food), then for maintenance at the rate of 1 every 3 days.

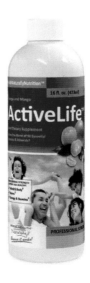
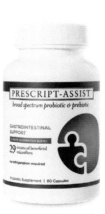

How to Supplement with Optional Nutrients

1st Line (Thiocyanate) Immune System Support Kit

1st Line (Thiocyanate) Immune System Support Kit offers an all-natural formulation that can equip the body to fight against a number of infections, as well as viruses. The patented formula was created by a British chemist and is made up of Thiocyanate Ions. When you add the formula to water, it creates a handy drink that forms the same molecules your body uses as its first line of defense to fight off yeast, fungi, germs, flu, viruses, and bacteria. 1st Line provides powerful protection against unwanted infection without harming the delicate balance of healthy bacteria in the body, an unfortunate side effect of using antibiotics. Even better, 1st Line is perfectly safe and convenient to use.

Ingredients:

- Sodium Thiocyanate 100ppm
- Sodium Hypothiocyanate 60ppm

Dosage:

Take 1 kit daily for 3 days (total of 3). 1st Line Kit should always be taken at least 90 minutes before and 90 minutes after food, approximately. 3 kits are the minimum and in serious conditions 10 kits over 10 days are best if finances allow. Take this to clear any infection which may be inside the cells.

Antarctic Pure Krill Oil

Krill, tiny crustaceans that resemble shrimp, can be found in the Southern Oceans. These are the only oceans around the world that are still unpolluted by heavy metal toxins that can now be found in many marketed fish oils. As a result, Krill are a supreme source of Omega 3, 6, and 9 fatty acids; they also provide protective antioxidant levels at three times higher than Vitamins A and E and 48 times greater than Omega 3 used in commercial fish oils. As a note, please consult with your physician before taking Krill or another fish dietary supplement if you have seafood allergies.

100% natural Neptune-source Antarctic Pure Krill Oil is made with a specialized formulation of Omega 3, 6, and 9 fatty acids, antioxidants, and other powerful ingredients to provide benefits like:

- Reduced heart/lung-damaging inflammation
- Better memory, concentration, and learning
- Balanced blood lipid and cholesterol levels
- Regulated blood sugar levels
- Improved joint health with decreased arthritic symptoms and associated pain
- Reduced effects of premature aging
- Protected cell membranes
- Healthier liver function
- Strengthened immune system
- Balanced moods
- Radiant skin health

Now Available as Vegetable Licap: Suitable for Vegetarians!

Ingredients:

Superba™ Krill Oil	1000mg
Phospholipids	450mg
Total Omega 3	250mg
EPA	120mg
DHA	70mg
Omega 6	15mg
Omega 9	80mg
Astaxanthin	110µg

Dosage:

Take 1 capsule, 2 times a day with food.

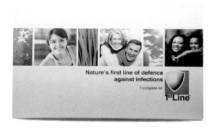

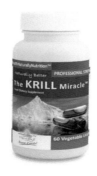

Naturally Better Vitamin E

Naturally Better Vitamin E is made with a self-emulsifying delivery system to offer consistent oral Tocotrienol absorption. It can provide benefits to support Alzheimer's disease, non-alcoholic fatty liver disease, cardiovascular health, stroke-related injuries, cholesterol reduction, immunity, hair growth, and especially cystic fibrosis.

Ingredients:

- Total d-Mixed-Tocotrienols (Tocomin∗) 20.00 mg
- Vitamin E Activity, IU 8.06 IU
- Plant Squalene 4.92 mg
- Phytosterol 1.72 mg

Dosage:

Take 1 capsule, 2 times a day.

Essential Digestive Plus™

The digestive system is an integrated system that affects all other systems throughout the body. Due to this unique interrelationship, it can be difficult to pinpoint the root cause of a digestive issue. Nonetheless, taking supportive digestive enzymes can help to alleviate a number of digestive problems.

The primary contributing factors to a number of diseases are yeast growth and incomplete digestion. Eating the right foods and taking the right nutritional supplements will provide little help if the digestive tract isn't fully equipped to break down and assimilate them. Supplementing with the right digestive enzymes is necessary to provide better absorption.

Proper absorption in the small intestine depends directly on beneficial digestive enzymes and highly absorbent surfaces. You can improve the function of the small intestine by addressing the underlying issues that could contribute to digestive imbalances and, ultimately, disease. Taking digestive enzymes can help to ease allergies and food intolerances. It will offer the support that the body needs while suffering from a lack of enzymes, low immunity, and excess sugar in the diet.

Ingredients:

FrutaFit® IQ Inulin	150mg
Protease SP Blend	82,000 HUT
Amylase	8,000 DU
Alpha Galactosidase	300 GLA
Glucoamylase	20 AGU
Lactase	1,000 ALU
Cellulase	600 CU
Invertase	525 INVU
Pectinase	55 endo PGU
Lipase	1,350 FIP

Dosage:

Take 1 capsule as you start your meals, 3 times per day.

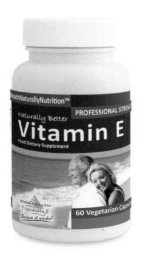
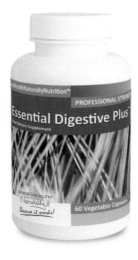

Understanding Acupressure

Stimulating an acupressure point located in the center of the chest will promote relaxation and improve breathing. You can safely and effectively stimulate the point with the **HealthPoint™** electro-acupressure kit. This kit is advantageous because it allows you to precisely locate the right acupuncture point and a number of other points to receive acupuncture benefits at home without using needles.

HealthPoint™ is painless, user-friendly, and entirely effective. The kit comes with an instructional DVD and book that provides information on more than 150 pain and non-pain health conditions that can be alleviated, including neck, back, joint, and headache issues.

Using systematic and gentle stimulation to target the body's natural healing system can expedite recovery in most cases. **HealthPoint™** offers a revolutionary technology developed by a leading pain control specialist, Dr. Julian Kenyon, 21 years ago. Today, you can use this innovative microchip technology to quickly and accurately target acupuncture points related to specific health issues, like the center chest point Cv17 to improve breathing.

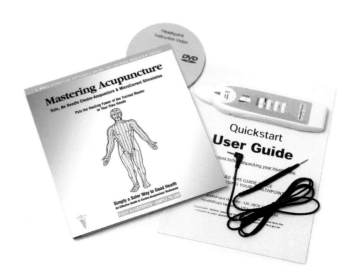

Conclusion:

Did you know that lung disease is the fourth leading cause of death?

1. **Heart disease**
2. **Cancer**
3. **Stroke**
4. **Lung disease**

Lung disease can better be understood as a lifestyle disease. This means that if you change your lifestyle, there is a great chance of partial or full recovery. When you implement the changes found in the 10 Step Plan, your body can naturally begin the healing process to recover your health.

‣ Drugs won't improve your health.

Drugs aren't effective since they can't make you healthy again. In a best case scenario, drugs may provide some relief. In a worst-case scenario, they will further damage your health and can even cause untimely death.

‣ This rehabilitation plan will always offer health improvements.

The worst outcome when using this plan will be that your health improves, but you still need to take some drugs if your health has been damaged irreparably by medication or a lung condition.

‣ Start slowly and begin rehabilitation step-by-step.

If you're not used to making major changes in your life, it may be difficult to adopt new healthy habits at first. But stick with it because...

‣ Your health is invaluable.

Robert Redfern, Your Health Coach

Let us know how you are doing by emailing feedback to:
robert@goodhealthhelpdesk.com

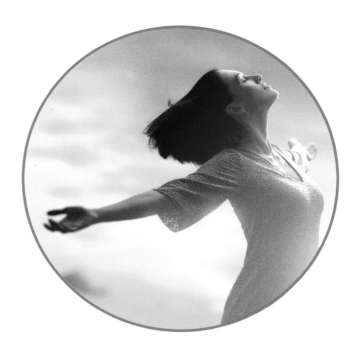

Daily Pulmonary Rehabilitation Plan

TIME	ACTION	AMOUNT

OPTIONAL ITEMS

TIME	ACTION	AMOUNT
Any time in the day on an empty stomach	Take 1st Line Immune System Support Kit	Take 1 kit daily for 3 days (total of 3). Take at least 90 minutes before and 90 minutes after food.
Before any cooked meal	Take Essential Digestive Plus™	Take 1 capsule, 3 times daily
With any meal	Take Naturally Better Vitamin E	Take 1 capsule, 2 times daily
With any meal	Take the Krill Miracle	Take 1 capsule, 2 times daily
For daily use alongside supplements	HealthPoint Kit	Use as appropriate on MicroCurrent stimulation points

BREAKFAST

TIME	ACTION	AMOUNT
After shower	Take Magnesium Oil Spray Ultra with OptiMSM®	Apply liberally across the chest, back and arm muscles
Before breakfast	Take Serranol	2 capsules, with water
With the Serranol®	Take D.I.P	1 capsule
Just before eating	Take Nascent Iodine Drops	4 drops in 25ml of water
With breakfast	Take ActiveLife 90	Take 15ml or ½ fl.oz in juice or water
With breakfast	Take Prescript Assist	1 capsule
Any time after breakfast	Take OxySorb drops	Hold 20 drops in the mouth
Any time after breakfast	Take Nascent Iodine Drops	4 drops in 25ml of water

LUNCH

TIME	ACTION	AMOUNT
Before any cooked meal	Take Serranol®	2 capsules, with water
With the Serranol®	Take D.I.P	1 capsule
Just before eating	Take Nascent Iodine Drops	4 drops in 25ml of water

EVENING MEAL

TIME	ACTION	AMOUNT
30 minutes before evening meal	Take Serranol®	2 capsules, with water
Just before eating	Take Nascent Iodine Drops	4 drops in 25ml of water
With the evening meal	Take Active Life 90	15ml or ½ fl.oz. in juice or water
With the evening meal	Take Prescript-Assist®	Take 1 capsule
Any time after the evening meal	Take OxySorb drops	Hold 20 drops in the mouth

All the books in this series:

Acne, Eczema & Psoriasis

Alzheimer's & Senility

Arthritis & Osteoporosis

Cancer: Breast, Colon, Pancreatic & Other Cancers

Cardiovascular Disease, PAD, Carotid & More

Chronic Fatigue, Fibromyalgia & Candida

Diabetes, Hypoglycemia, & Cholesterol Healthy Levels

Electro-Acupressure – Self-Treatment of the Acu Points

Fertility Problems

Heart Disease, Angina, Valves & More

High & Low Blood Pressure

IBS, Crohn's, Colitis, Ulcers & Other Digestive Problems

Lung Disease, COPD, Emphysema & More

Macular Degeneration, Cataracts & Diabetic Retinopathy

Men: Prostate, EDF, & Hormones

MS, RA, Lupus, Psoriatic Arthritis & Other Auto Immune Diseases

Stress & Anxiety

Stroke Recovery & Prevention

Women: PMS, Menopause, Fibroids, PCOS & Fibroids

Other Books by Robert Redfern:

The 'Miracle Enzyme' is Serrapeptase

Turning A Blind Eye

Mastering Acupuncture

EquiHealth Equine Acupressure

ABOUT THIS BOOK

Robert Redfern - Your Personal Health Coach

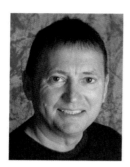

Robert Redfern is a passionate health coach that strives to offer you the best information and tools so that you can become a natural health expert to support you and your family's health.

This book combines all of Robert's work and research on lung health into a user-friendly Pulmonary Rehabilitation Plan that can be used for naturally improved health.

For more information, you can consult the Naturally Healthy Publications website for dedicated Good Health Coaching from Robert Redfern.

Please visit **www.NaturallyHealthyPublications.com** today to find more information on lung health conditions related to:

- COPD
- Emphysema
- Bronchitis
- Fibrosis
- Bronchiectasis
- Cystic Fibrosis
- Cough - Chronic
- Bronchial Asthma
- Pneumoconiosis, Asbestosis & Dust Conditions

"I could hardly believe the improvement in his health. We were on a 3 week cruise and met one of the other passengers, obviously in poor health. His lips were blue and his breathing laboured. When we got off to visit places he could hardly walk. He was 72 years old and told us he suffered from asbestosis, emphysema and heart problems."

"Having used your formulation for all my family and friends, I just had to tell him about it. I happened to have a spare bottle with me, so I gave it to him. He took 3 per day for the rest of the cruise, and even I could hardly believe the improvement in his health. By the end of the cruise, his lips were pink and he was able to do the full excursions. I have spoken to him since and he has bought some himself and is now able to drive for the first time in a long time."

Mrs. Hardman

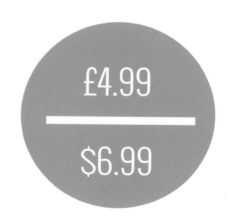

£4.99
—
$6.99

If you need help, please visit **www.GoodHealthHelpDesk.com** and ask questions there.

Let us know how you are doing by emailing feedback to: **robert@goodhealthhelpdesk.com**

Printed in Great Britain
by Amazon

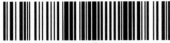